TERRANCE
THE HOTHEAD

A BOOK TO HELP CHILDREN MANAGE BIG FEELINGS

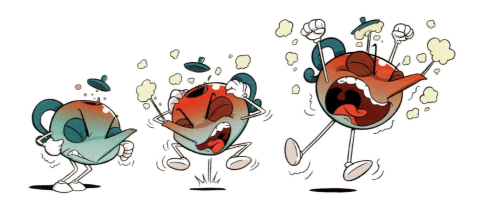

Written by **LISA CLOHERTY, MS, CCC-SLP**
Illustrated by **ALEX LOPEZ**

Published by ASHA Press

An imprint of the American Speech-Language-Hearing Association (ASHA)

The American Speech-Language-Hearing Association (ASHA) is the national professional, scientific, and credentialing association for audiologists; speech-language pathologists; speech, language, and hearing scientists; audiology and speech-language pathology support personnel; and students. ASHA works to promote the interests of these professionals and to advocate for people with communication disorders.

The opinions contained herein are the views of the contributors and are not to be construed as reflecting official policies or recommendations of ASHA.

No use of this material—including translation, storage in a retrieval system, microfilming, recording, or posting to any site or page on the World Wide Web, or otherwise—is allowed without written permission from the publisher.

Copyright ©2022, American Speech-Language-Hearing Association
Illustration copyright ©2022, Alex Lopez

ISBN: 978-1-58041-279-7

Copies may be ordered from:

ASHA Product Sales
2200 Research Boulevard
Rockville, MD 20850-3289
Tel: 888-498-6699
Fax: 301-296-8590
www.asha.org

ASHA Content Consultant: Diane Paul, PhD, CCC-SLP, CAE
Product Manager: Catharine Gray
Art Director: Emerald Ong

Printed in the U.S.A.

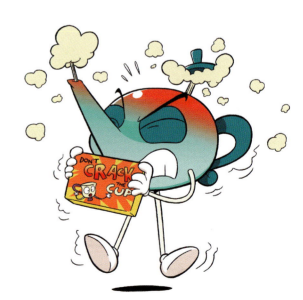

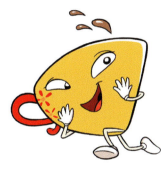

To Owen, who inspires me to
live and love fiercely every single day.

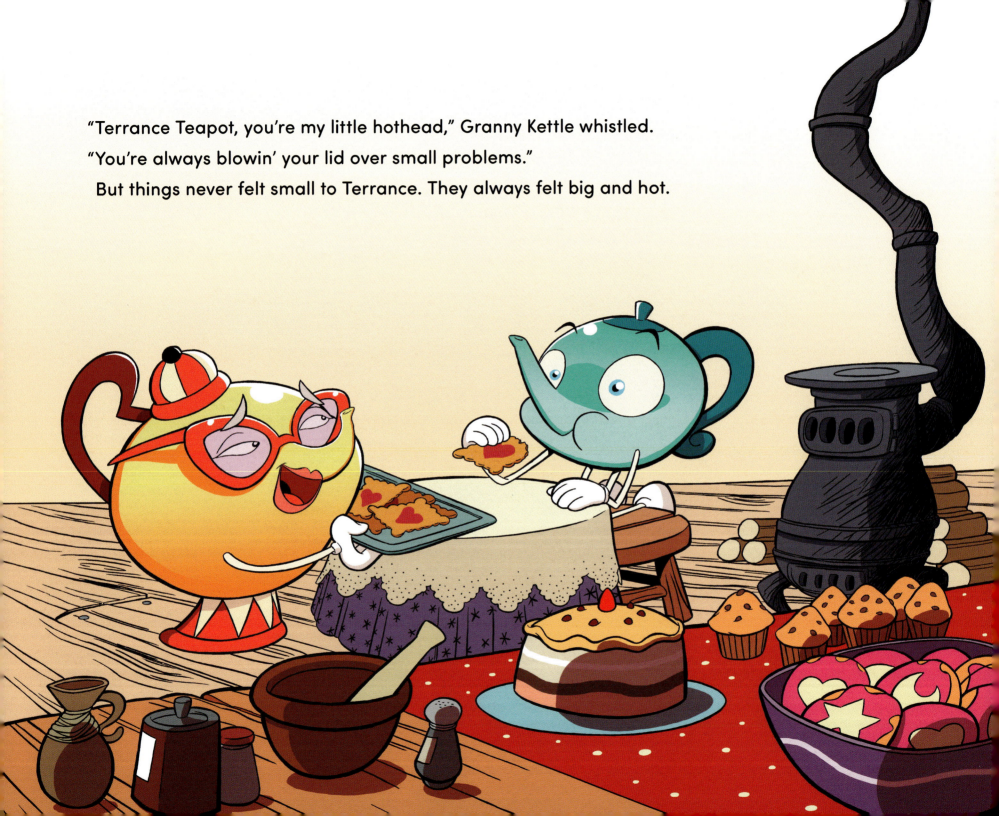

"Terrance Teapot, you're my little hothead," Granny Kettle whistled.

"You're always blowin' your lid over small problems."

But things never felt small to Terrance. They always felt big and hot.

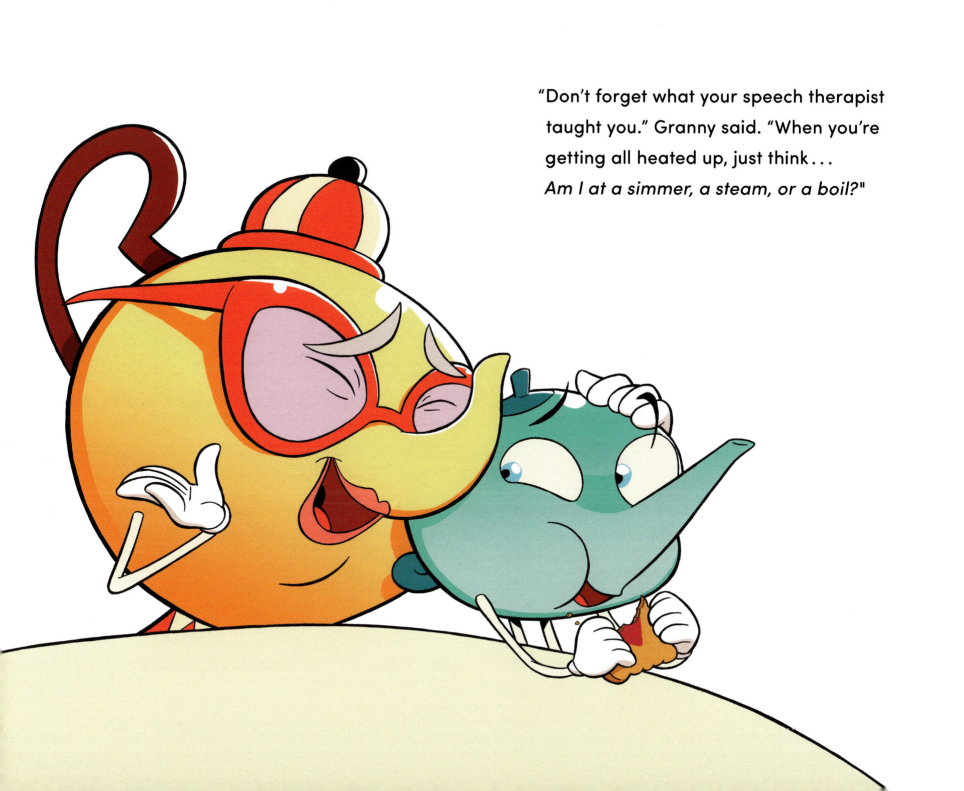

"Don't forget what your speech therapist taught you." Granny said. "When you're getting all heated up, just think...
Am I at a simmer, a steam, or a boil?"

At recess, Coach Ice organized a game of tea-ball. Terrance rattled with excitement.

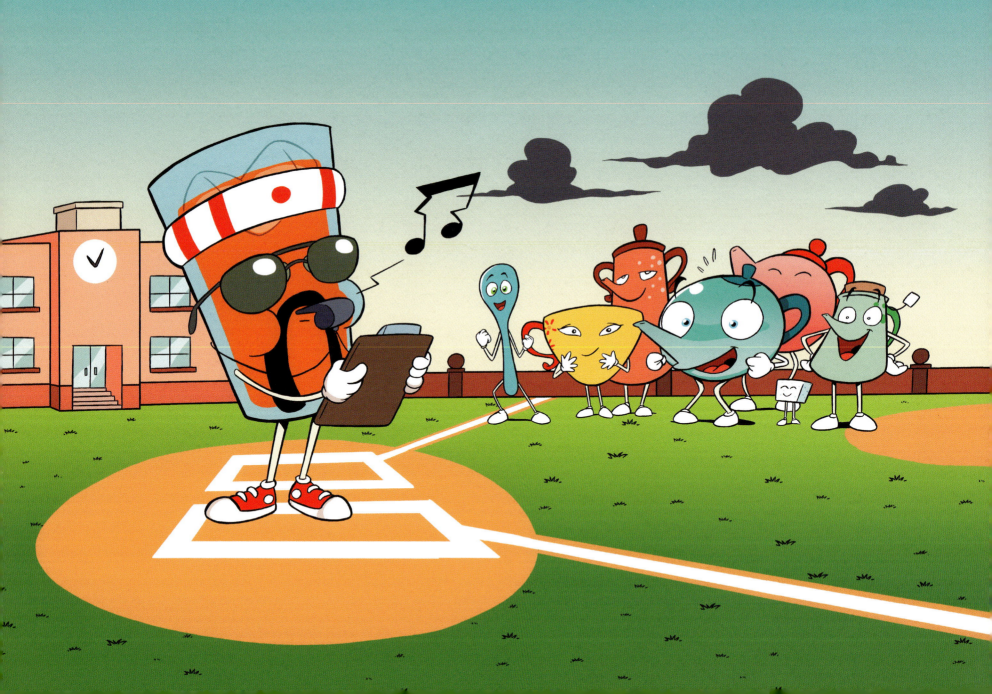

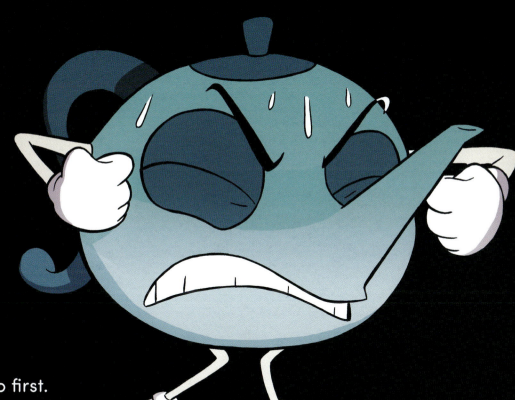

Terrance wanted to go first.
Terrance needed to go first.
Terrance absolutely **HAD** to go first.

"First up is Lanie Cup," Coach called.
Terrance felt big and hot.
"That is not fair!" Terrance wailed.

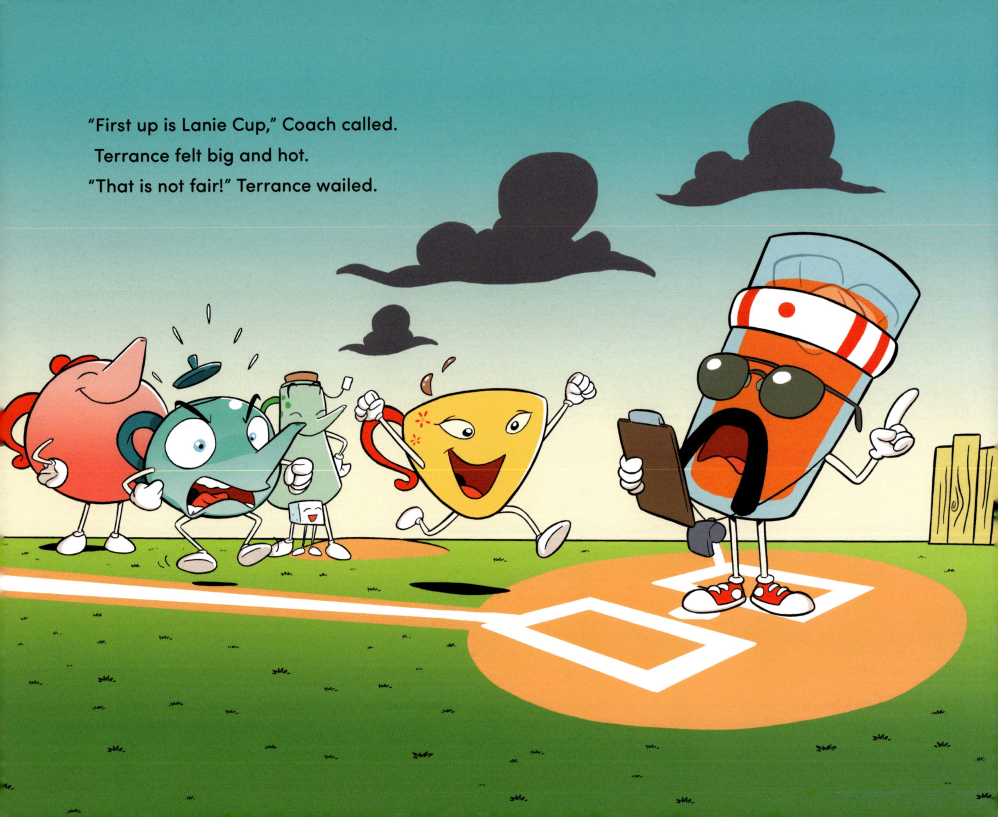

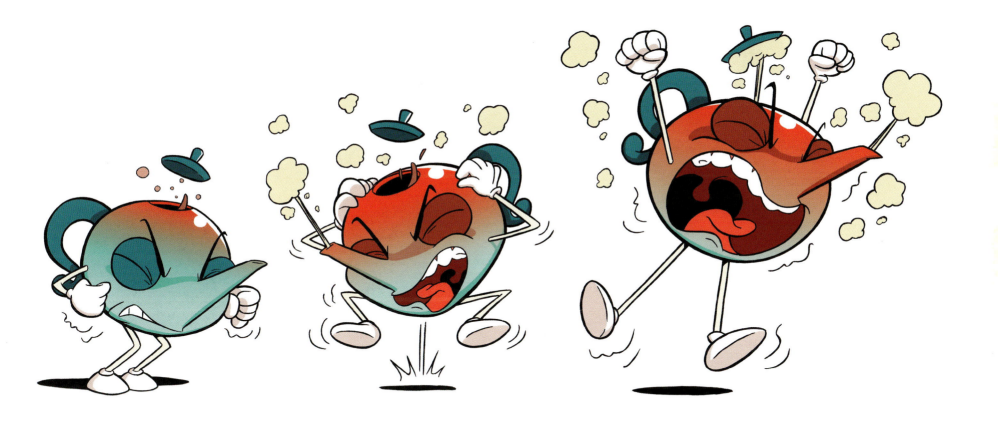

Terrance bubbled and hissed... smashed and crashed... and then he **EXPLODED!**

Coach Ice came over. "Are you at a simmer, a steam, or a boil?"
Terrance was too boiling to speak.

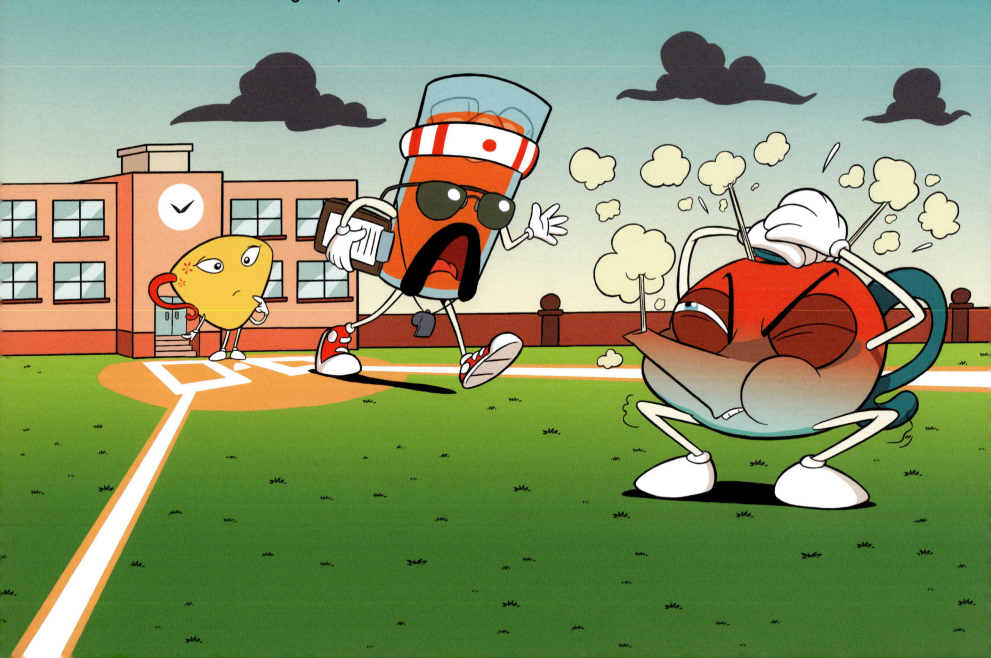

"Count 10 breaths," Coach Ice said.

Terrance closed his eyes and breathed out slowly.

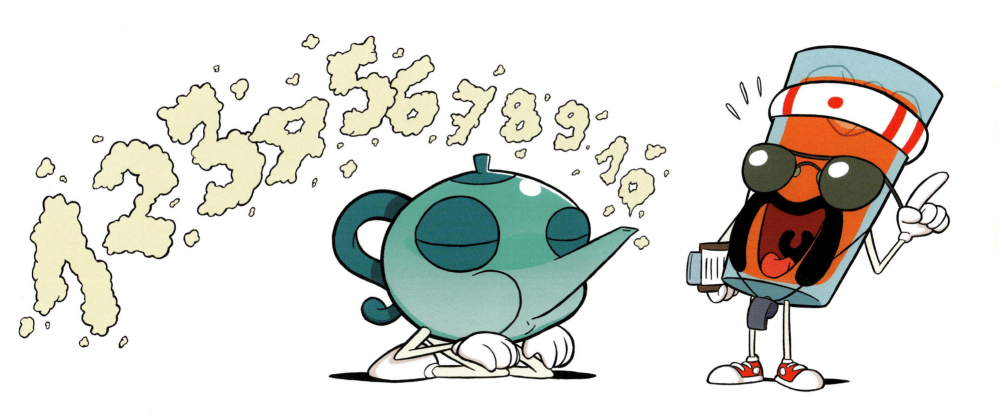

"Great job cooling down. Now let's get back on the field."

Back in class, Lanie sat next to Terrance. "Hey Terrance, want to hear a joke?" Lanie clinked. Terrance groaned, "Not another teapot joke."

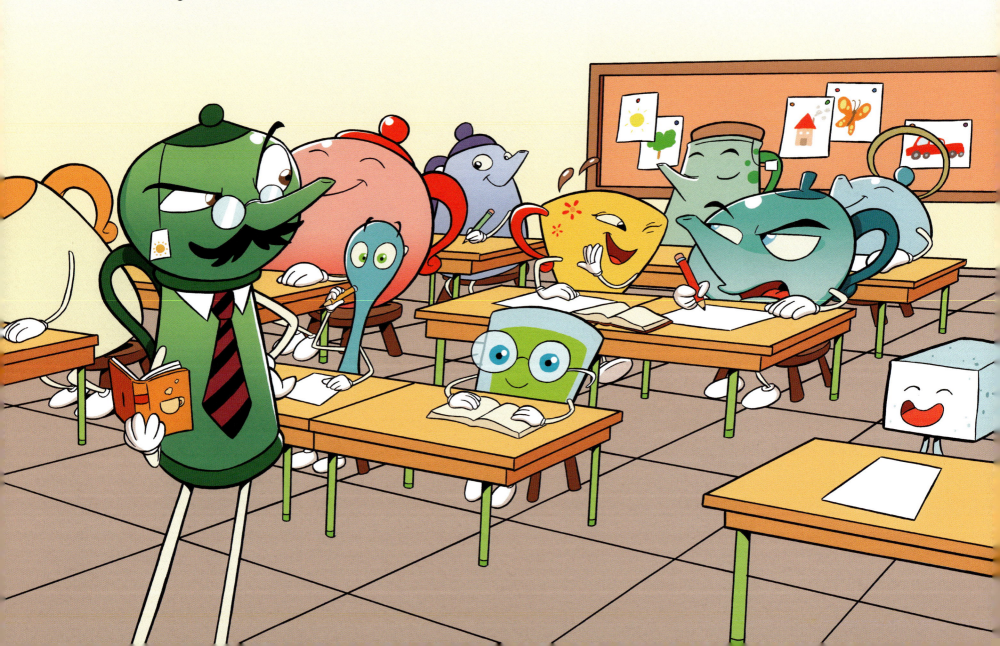

Lanie didn't listen. "Why do teapots always get in trouble?" Terrance felt big and hot. "Because they're naugh-tea," Lanie laughed.

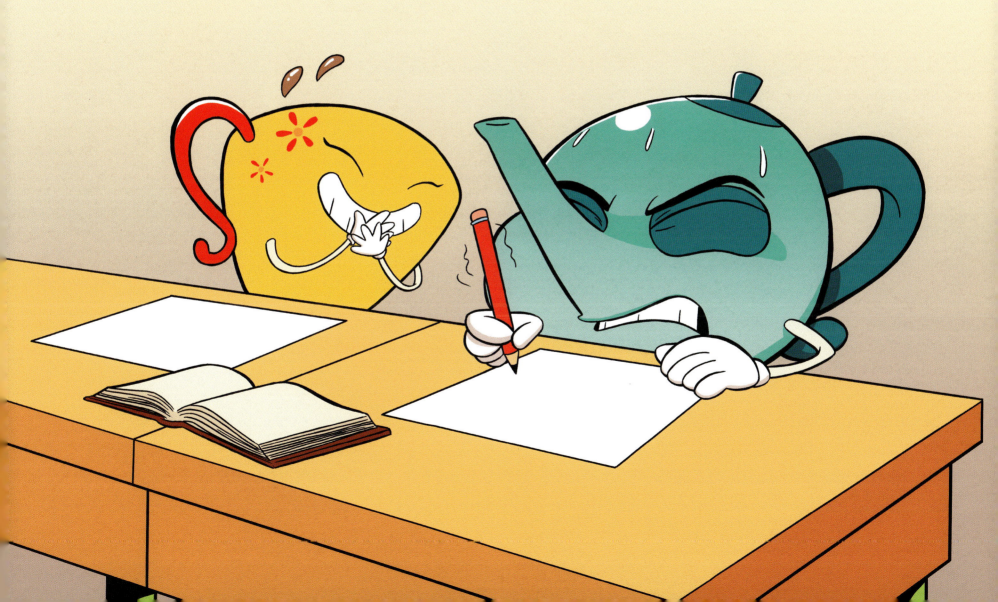

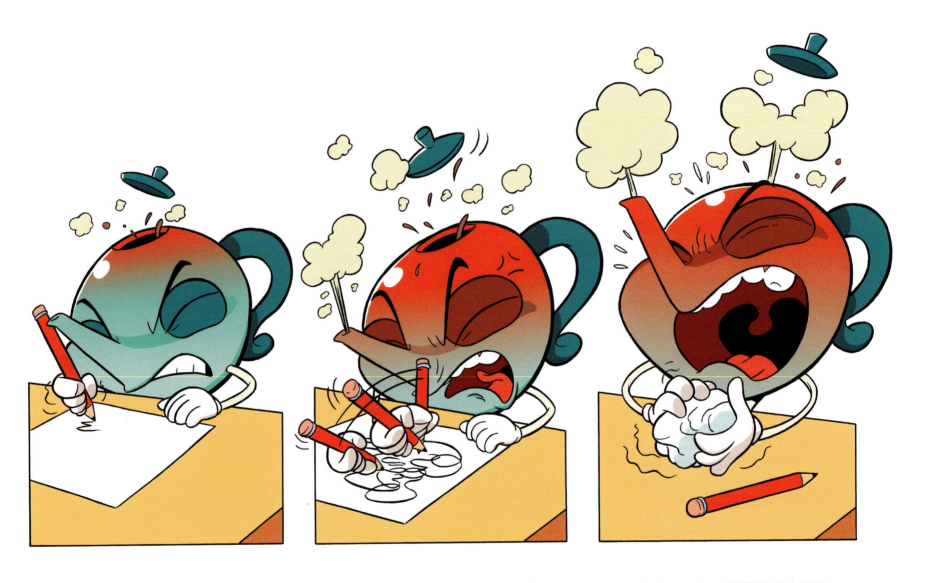

Terrance huffed and puffed... whistled and screeched... and then he EXPLODED!

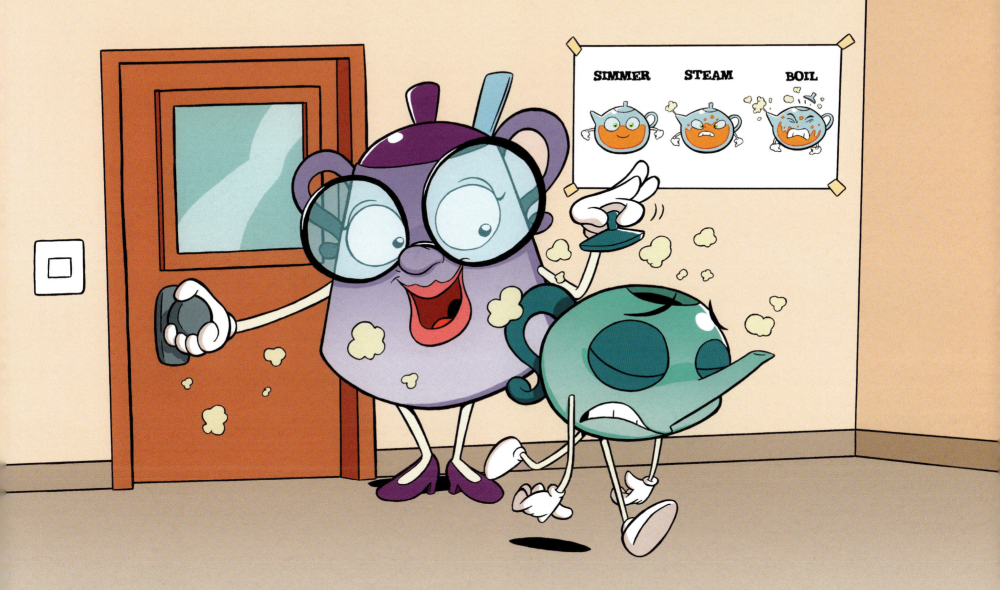

Terrance went to visit Lady Grey's office.

"How you feelin' sugar?" she asked sweetly. "Let's open your lid and cool down. Are you at a simmer, a steam, or a boil?"

Terrance sighed. Sometimes it was hard to tell.

"A steam, I think," he finally mumbled.

Lady Grey smiled, "Why do you think Lanie is always telling you jokes?"

She's tea-sing me, Terrance thought at first.

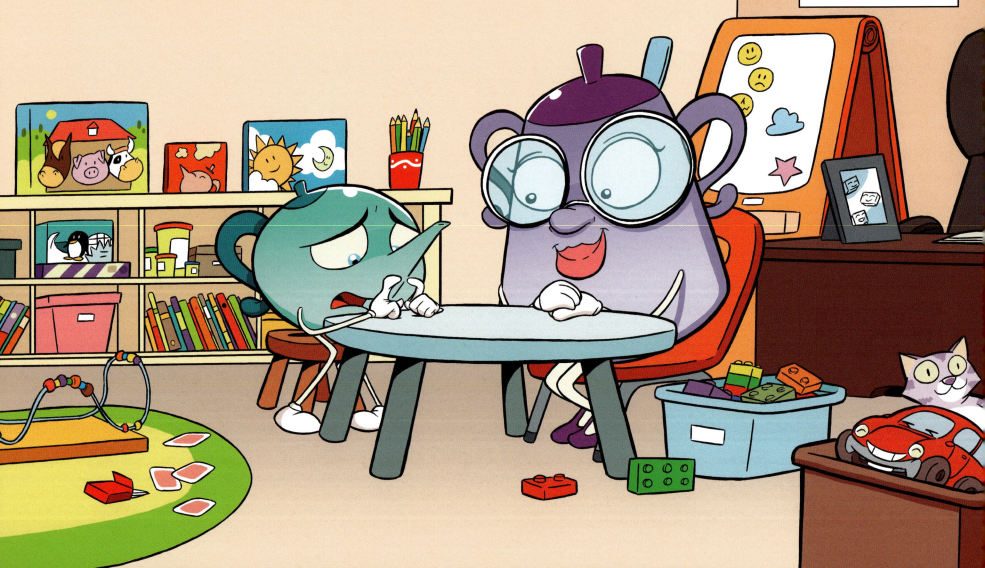

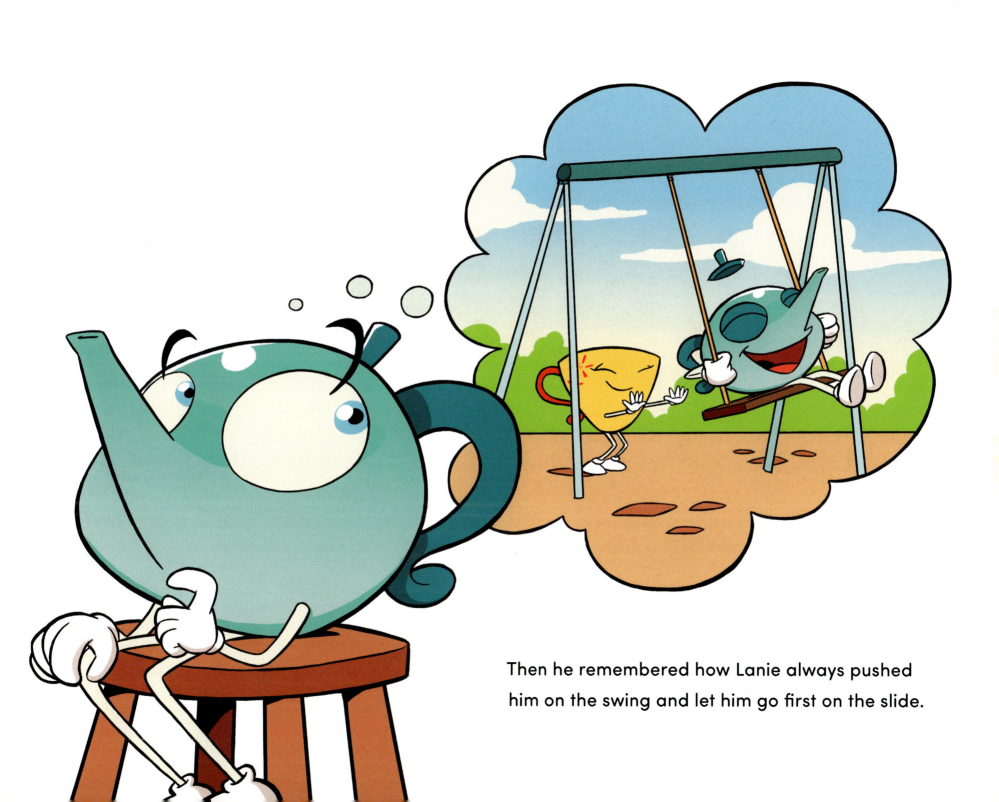

Then he remembered how Lanie always pushed him on the swing and let him go first on the slide.

"Maybe," Terrance said, "she wants to be my friend."

"Great thinking!" Lady Grey cheered.

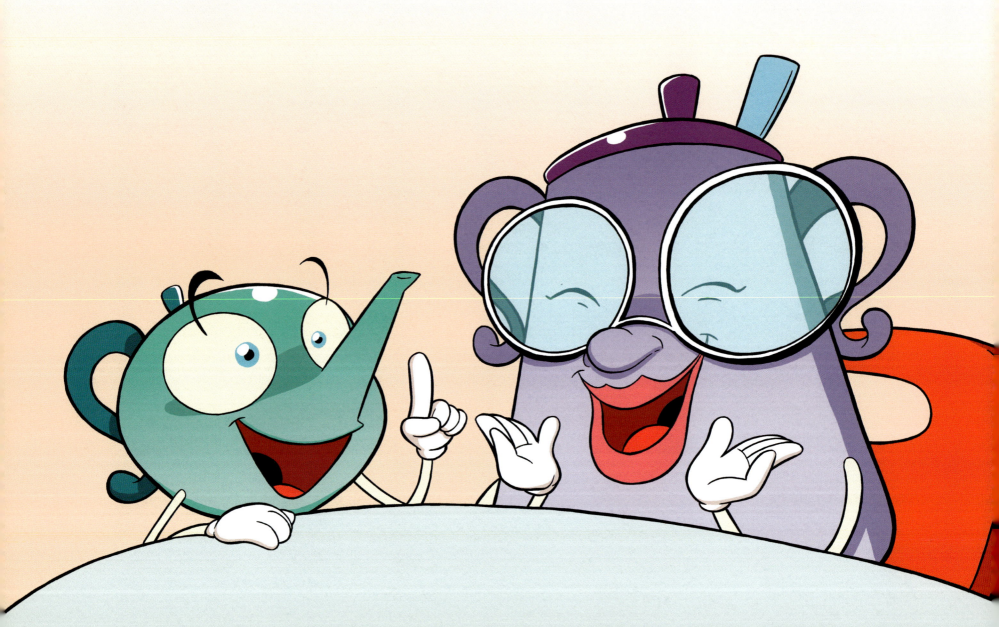

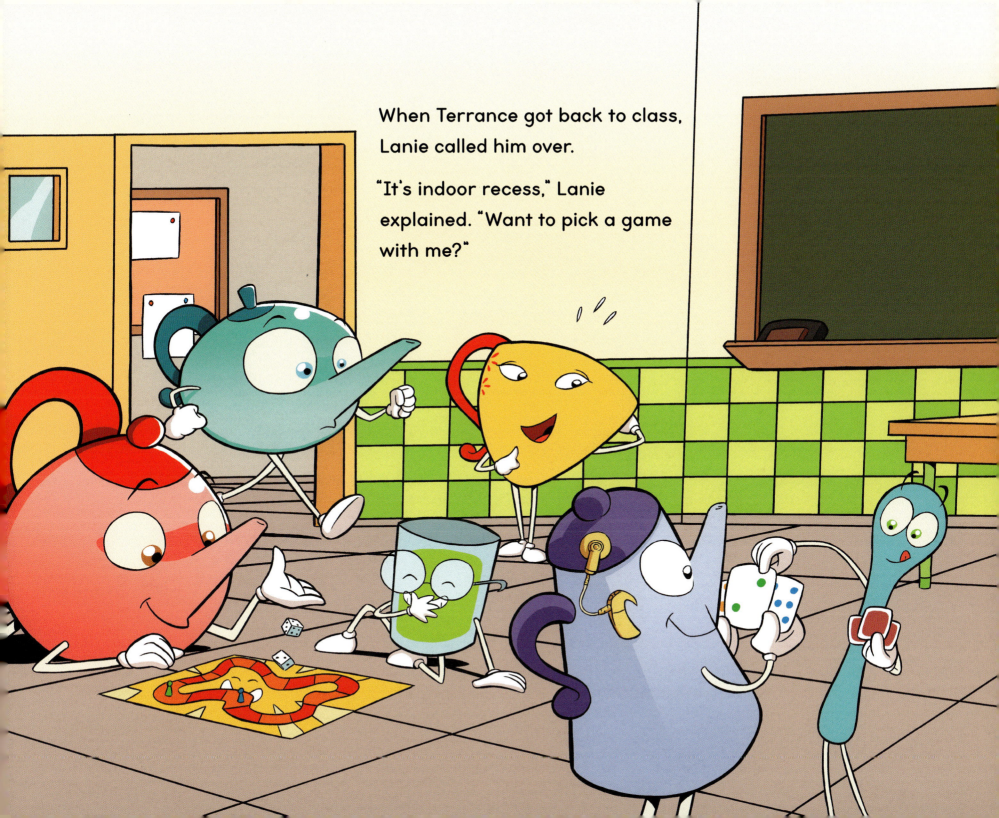

When Terrance got back to class, Lanie called him over.

"It's indoor recess," Lanie explained. "Want to pick a game with me?"

"Let's play Don't Crack the Cup," Terrance declared.

"Nah, that game is not my cup of tea," Lanie said. "I like Pretty Pretty Teapot."

Terrance whined, "I am not playing Pretty Pretty Teapot!"

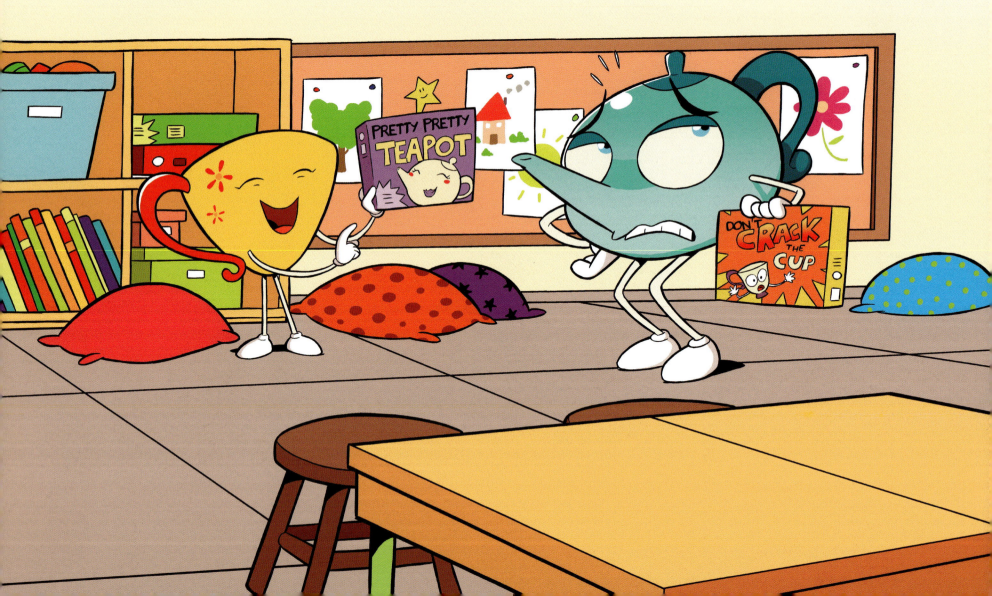

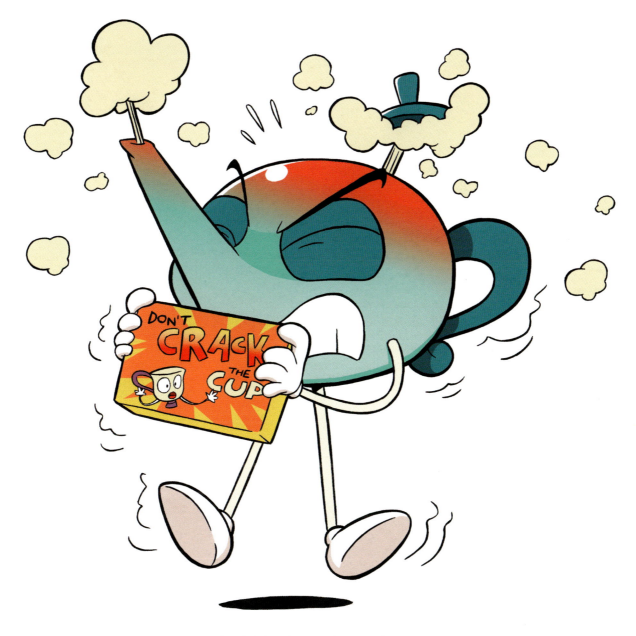

Terrance felt big and hot again.   He bubbled and hissed...   whistled and screeched...

. . . but just before he exploded, he thought about how much he'd like to be Lanie's friend.

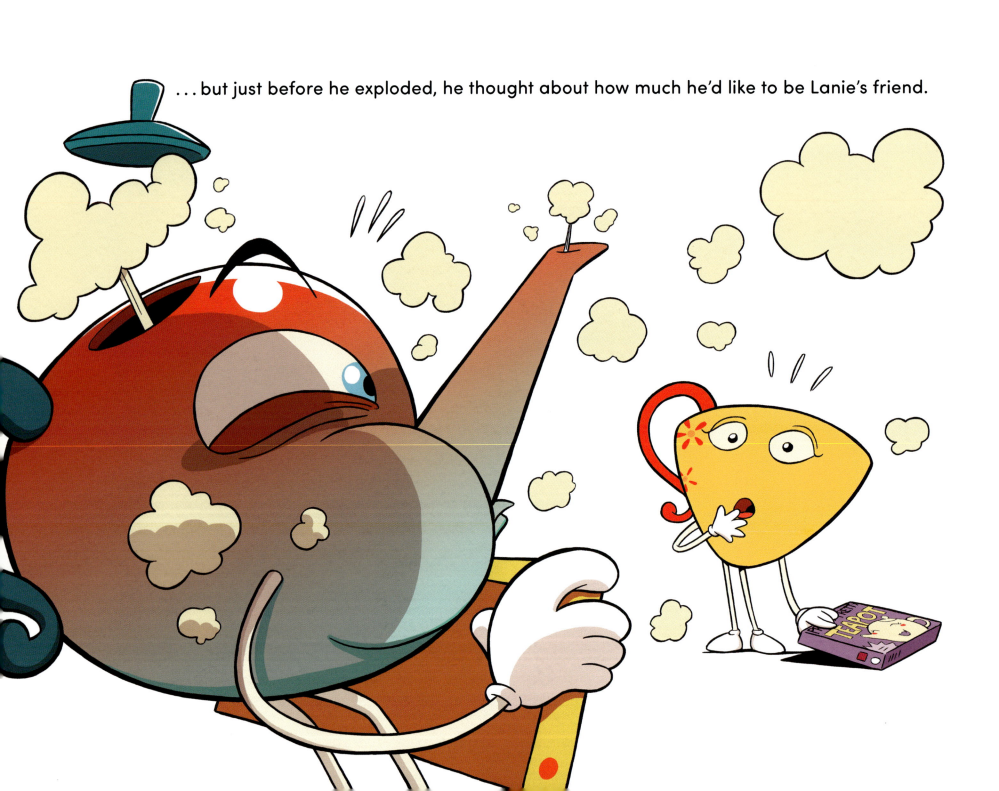

Terrance took a deep breath and slowly, slowly, slowly cooled

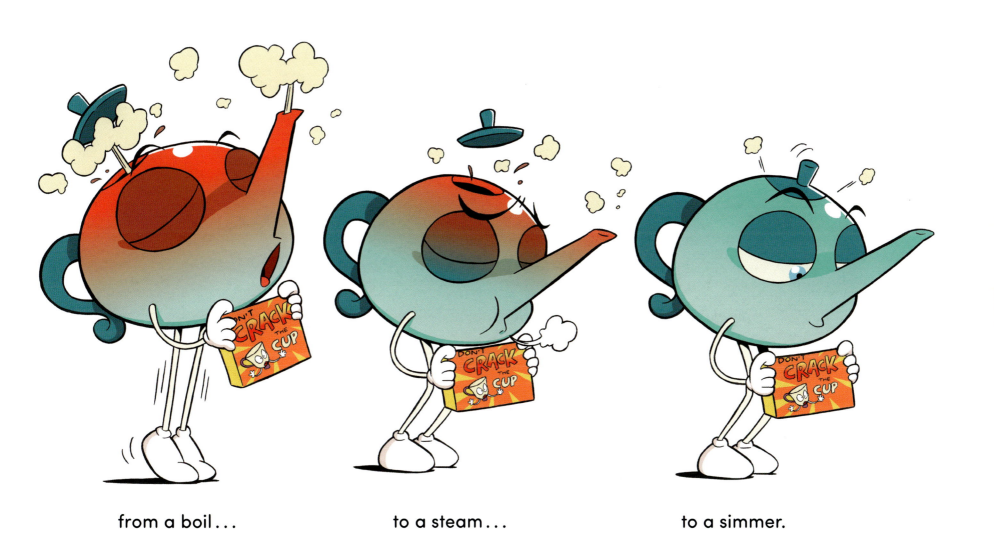

from a boil...   to a steam...   to a simmer.

He realized with great delight that he felt much better.

"Why don't we play Pretty Pretty Teapot first," Terrance suggested, "and Don't Crack the Cup after?"

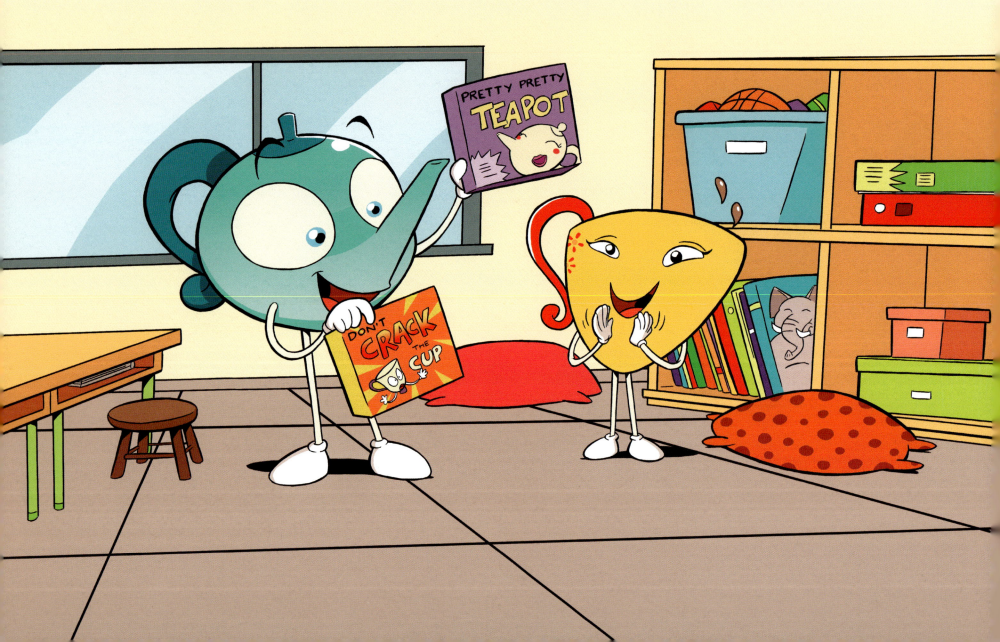

Just before they began to play, Terrance turned to Lanie.

"What kind of dinosaur loves to drink tea?" Terrance asked. She smiled and shrugged.

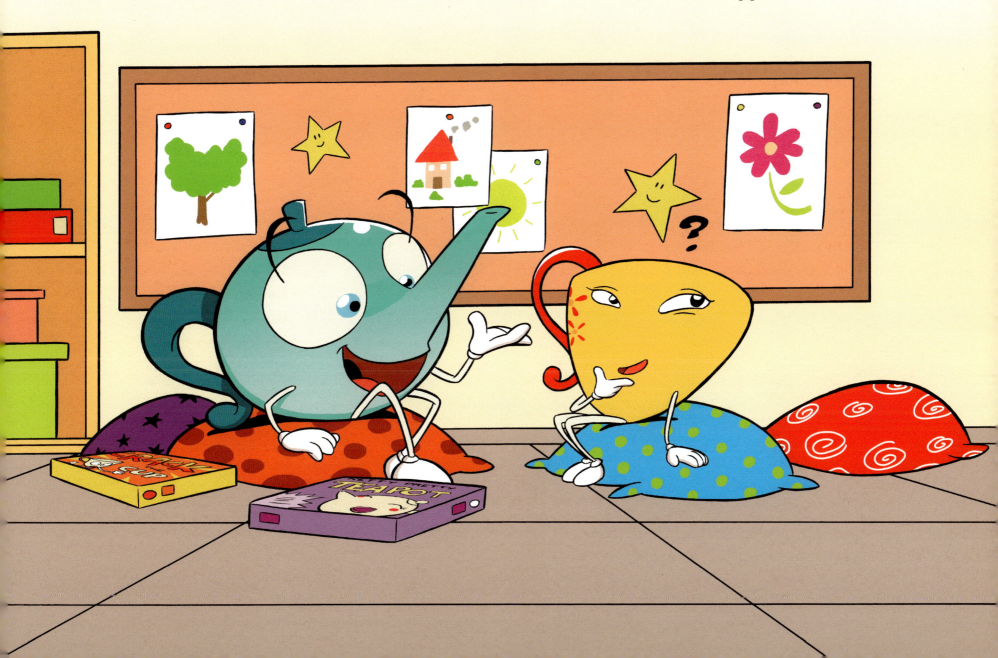

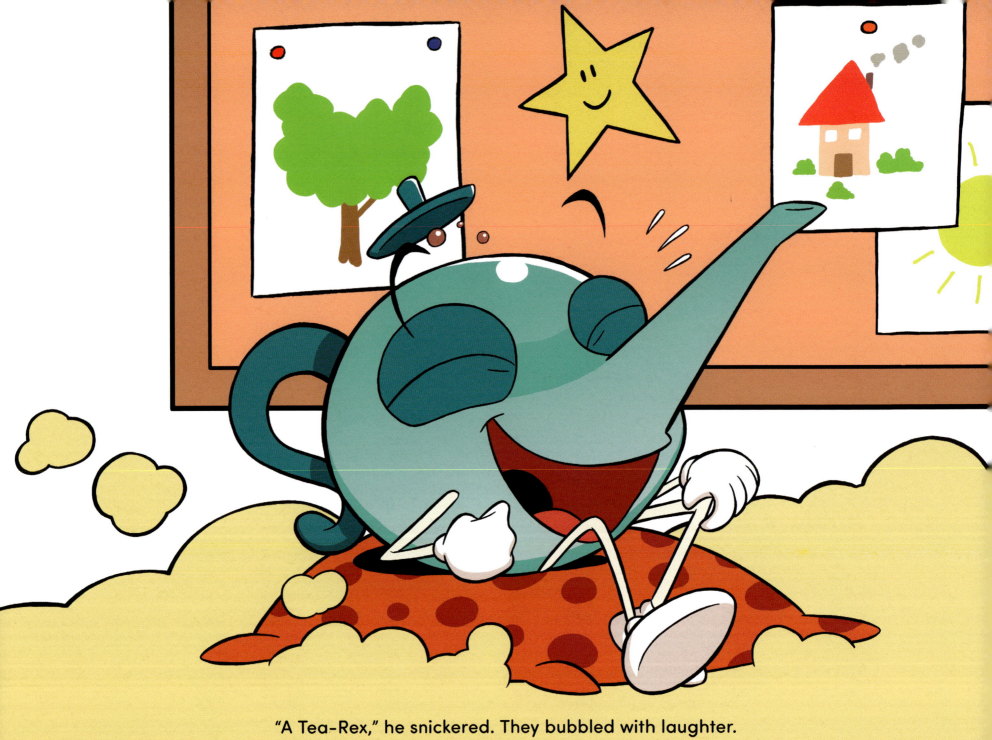

"A Tea-Rex," he snickered. They bubbled with laughter.

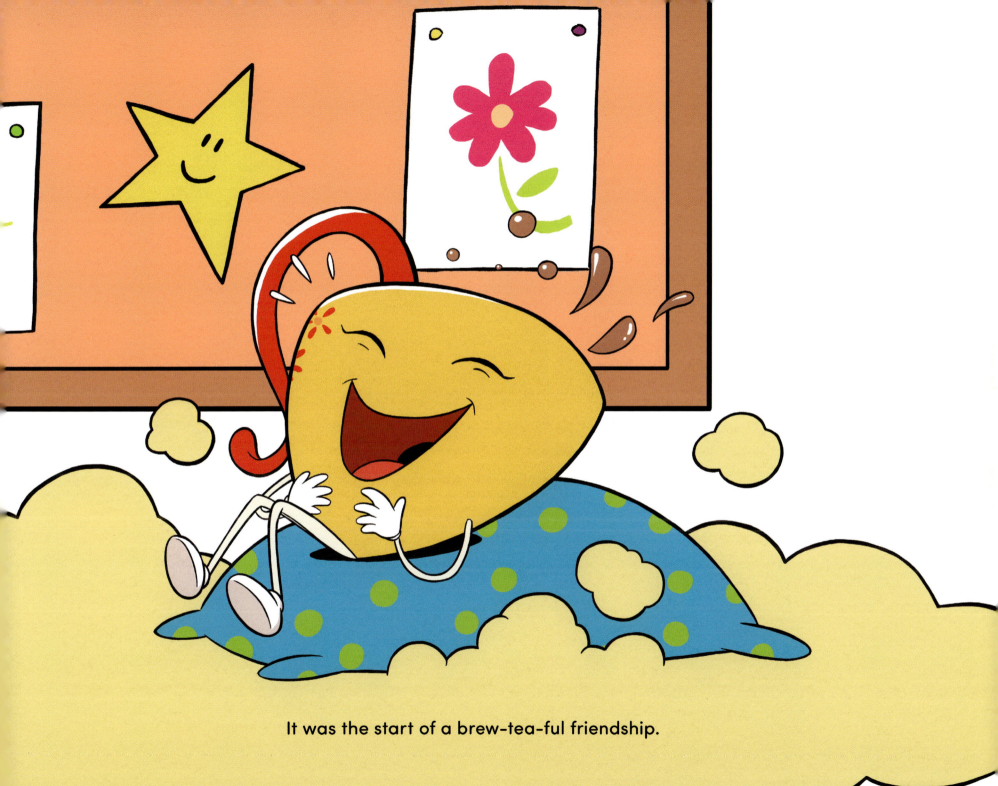

It was the start of a brew-tea-ful friendship.

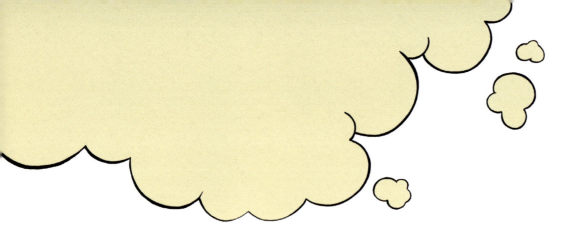
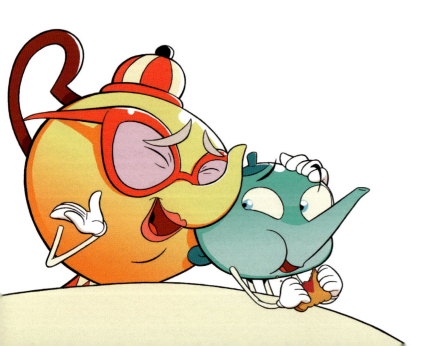

INTRODUCTION

Over the last few years, several programs—such as Yale's Center for Emotional Intelligence and Michelle Garcia Winner's Social Thinking Program—have helped bring emotional identification and emotional regulation curricula to our schools. Speech-language pathologists, as well as other professionals, use these programs to help students in all aspects of social-emotional functioning.

Speech-language pathologists work with children who struggle to identify and regulate their emotions. Helping with emotional regulation and communication can impact how children relate to others and create meaningful friendships.

Terrance has big reactions to small problems. He has difficulty identifying his emotions and calming down. *Terrance the Hothead* provides the language for these emotions and incorporates abstract language (e.g., perspective taking, idioms) to enhance social skills instruction.

Terrance the Hothead can be used by speech-language pathologists, occupational therapists, social workers, guidance counselors, teachers, and parents as an introduction to or reinforcement of social training programs. Educators and parents can use the terms *simmer, steam,* and *boil* to cue children during moments of frustration.

TERRANCE—KEY TERMS

Studies suggest that when young children are introduced to exercises that intentionally build their emotional intelligence it has a positive impact on their social interaction, emotional identification, and self-regulation. These aspects of social-emotional development are crucial in helping children experience positive relationships and build friendships. Strong social-emotional skills have a powerful impact on academic performance, outlook on life, career paths, and a child's health. Good communication skills can help children identify and regulate their emotions.

Emotional Identification
The ability to recognize and understand feelings and how they impact actions/behaviors. (e.g., Terrance is excited to play "tea-ball.")

Perspective Taking
The ability to identify and understand another person's feelings and how our actions affect how the other person feels. (e.g., Lanie wants to be Terrance's friend, so she tells him teapot jokes.)

Emotional Regulation
The ability to identify and express emotions in socially appropriate ways. Emotional regulation allows us to be flexible enough to delay reactions and behaviors as needed. Emotional regulation skills can help us learn to calm down and control our behavior when we feel angry, frustrated, or excited. (e.g., Terrance feels frustrated when Lanie wants to play a game that he doesn't like. Instead of getting angry, Terrance suggests that they take turns.)

QUESTIONS

Use these questions to help children relate to the emotional development of the characters in the book.

1. *Idioms* are phrases that say one thing but mean something different (e.g., "raining cats and dogs"). What do the following idioms mean?
   - blowing your lid
   - getting heated up
   - boiling over
   - cooling down
2. Name some examples of small problems. Name some examples of big problems.
3. What is a small reaction? What is a big reaction?
4. Did Terrance's reaction match the size of his problem?
5. How did Terrance try to cool down? Did it work?
6. What are some fair ways to decide who goes first?
7. What is the difference between laughing at you and laughing with you?
8. What three things did Lanie do to show Terrance she wanted to be his friend?
9. What can you say/do if you want to make a new friend?
10. What does *compromise* mean? How did Terrance compromise?

BONUS: Can you think of a silly joke?

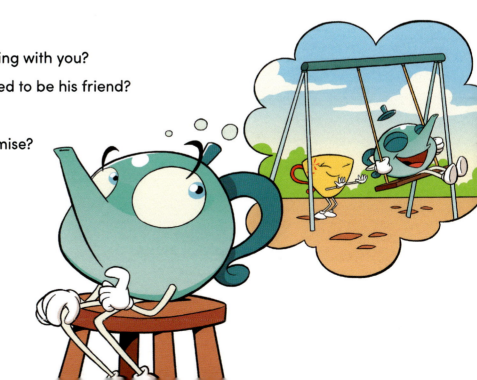

EMOTIONS PRACTICE

In *Terrance the Hothead,* Terrance displays emotions that range from excitement to frustration. Read the situations below, and answer how you might feel.

1. Your brother borrows your bike and breaks the basket. How would you feel?
2. You hear thunder and lightning when you're trying to sleep. How would you feel?
3. Your best friend is moving to a new school. How would you feel?
4. You win first prize at the science fair. How would you feel?
5. Your family throws you a surprise party. How would you feel?

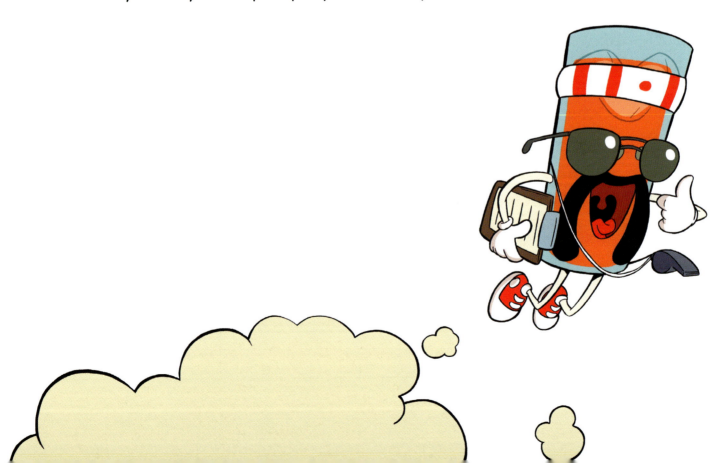

WORKSHEET

Use these strategies to help your child respond to a challenging situation. When we stop to cool down, we make better choices, have better friendships, and feel better about ourselves.

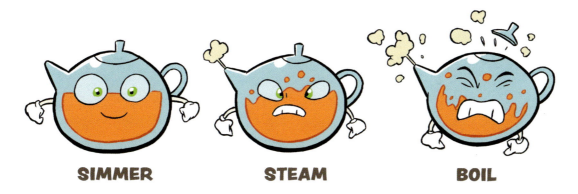

SIMMER **STEAM** **BOIL**

1. Something happens (e.g., You don't get to go first)
2. Pause and think about how you are feeling. What word describes how you feel? (e.g., *frustrated*)
3. Take a break before you act.
4. If you are feeling boiling hot:
   - step away,
   - take a deep breath,
   - count to 10,
   - talk to a trusted grownup, and
   - think about something that makes you happy or calm.
5. Once you've cooled from a boil, to a steam, to a simmer, give it another try!

SOCIAL-EMOTIONAL MILESTONES

Listed below are some developmental milestones related to a child's social-emotional development (up to age 7 years). It is important to remember that each child develops at their own pace given their specific learning and developmental needs. If you are concerned about your child's social-emotional development, you may want to connect with a speech-language pathologist.

18 months

- Needs help coping with temper tantrums.
- Engages in simple pretend play such as feeding a baby doll.
- Demonstrates joint attention—for example, pointing to a toy and looking to an adult to see if they notice, too.
- Acknowledges others by making eye contact or vocalizing.

2 years

- Plays side by side near children (parallel play). Occasionally includes other children.
- Shows increased independence and may say "no" often.
- Gets excited about the company of others and shows some separation anxiety.
- Acts out in frustration when unable to verbalize feelings.

3 years

- Shows empathy and kindness to others.
- Takes turns in games and is learning to share.
- Feels unsure about new places or routines at times.
- Greets others without having to be reminded to do so.

4 years

- Cooperates in play with other children.
- Engages in pretend play, linking two or more connected ideas.
- Understands that emotions change in different situations.
- Begins to tell jokes.

5–6 years

- Agrees to following rules and to cooperating.
- Uses imagination to create stories.
- Discusses emotions and feelings.
- Recognizes another person's need for help.

6–7 years

- Shows awareness of one's own and others' emotions.
- Begins to develop self-control.
- Feels hurt when called names.
- Draws emotional stability from interactions with familiar adults.

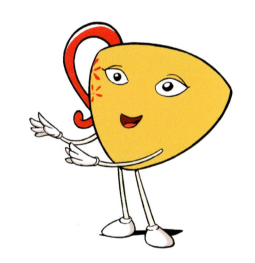

REFERENCES

Milestones are from the following two sources.

- Kipping, P., Gard, A., Gilman, L., & Gorman, J. (2012). *Speech and language development chart* (3rd ed.). Pro-Ed.
- U.S. Department of Education. (2015). *Milestones: Understanding your child's social and emotional development from birth to age 5.* https://www.electronic-therapy.com/wp-content/uploads/2019/08/Social-and-Emotional-Development-0-5.pdf

ACKNOWLEDGMENTS

I would like to thank my husband for being my constant supporter, sounding board, and for all your silly Terrance adventures over dinner. My two beautiful children—Maya and Owen—who encourage me to follow my dreams. Thank you to the ASHA staff members who believed in this story. I am forever grateful for your dedication and support throughout this process.

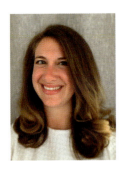

ABOUT THE AUTHOR

Lisa Cloherty, MS, CCC-SLP, is a pediatric speech-language pathologist and a children's book author. She loves puns and silly jokes almost as much as she loves mint tea. She is also the author of *Katie Spector the Art Collector* by Charming Books Press. Most of Lisa's stories revolve around community and acceptance of children with differing abilities. Lisa lives in Connecticut with her husband and two children. You can find out more about Lisa's upcoming books at www.lisaclohertybooks.com.

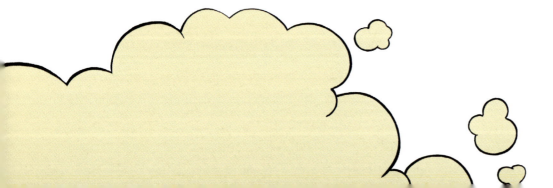

ABOUT THE ILLUSTRATOR

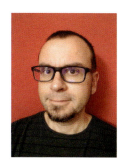

Alex Lopez is from Sabadell, Spain. He became a professional illustrator and comic-book artist in 2001, but he's been drawing ever since he can remember. Lopez's pieces have been published in many countries, including the United States, United Kingdom, Spain, France, Italy, Belgium, and Turkey. He's worked on a variety of projects from illustrated books to video games to marketing pieces.

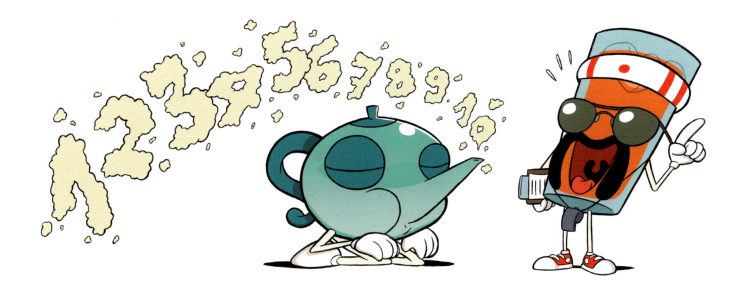